Healthy Choices

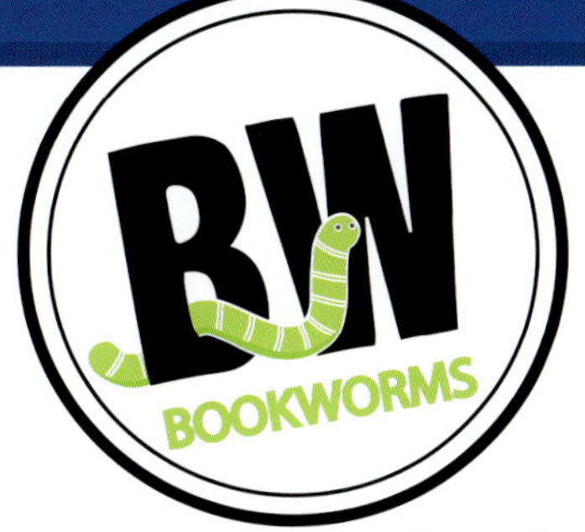

GOING TO THE DOCTOR

By R. J. MacReady

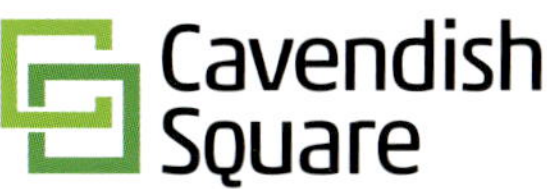

New York

Published in 2022 by Cavendish Square Publishing, LLC
243 5th Avenue, Suite 136, New York, NY 10016

First Edition

Website: cavendishsq.com

Library of Congress Cataloging-in-Publication Data

Names: MacReady, R. J., author.
Title: Going to the doctor / R.J. MacReady.
Description: First. | New York : Cavendish Square Publishing, [2022] |
Series: Healthy choices | Includes index.
Identifiers: LCCN 2020034873 | ISBN 9781502659682 (library binding) | ISBN 9781502659668 (paperback) | ISBN 9781502659675 (set) | ISBN 9781502659699 (ebook)
Subjects: LCSH: Children–Medical examinations–Juvenile literature. | Children–Preparation for medical care–Juvenile literature.
Classification: LCC RJ50.5 .M33 2022 | DDC 618.92/0075–dc23
LC record available at https://lccn.loc.gov/2020034873

Editor: Greg Roza
Designer: Andrea Davison-Bartolotta

The photographs in this book are used by permission and through the courtesy of: Cover Studio Romantic/Shutterstock.com; p. 5 Tim Kitchen/DigitalVision/Getty Images; p. 7 Thomas Northcut/DigitalVision/Getty Images; p. 9 andresr/E+/Getty Images; p. 11 FS Productions/Getty Images; p. 13 Lordn/iStock/Getty Images Plus/Getty Images; p. 15 FatCamera/E+/Getty Images; p. 17 Ariel Skelley/DigitalVision/Getty Images; pp. 19, 21 SDI Productions/E+/Getty Images; p. 23 monkeybusinessimages/iStock/Getty Images Plus/Getty Images.

CPSIA compliance information: Batch #CW22CSQ: For further information contact Cavendish Square Publishing LLC, New York, New York, at 1-877-980-4450.

Printed in the United States of America

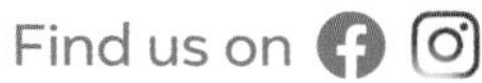

CONTENTS

Health Helpers

Doctors care about your health. They want you to feel good and be well! They go to school for many years. They know what to do when you're sick or hurt. They help people make healthy choices.

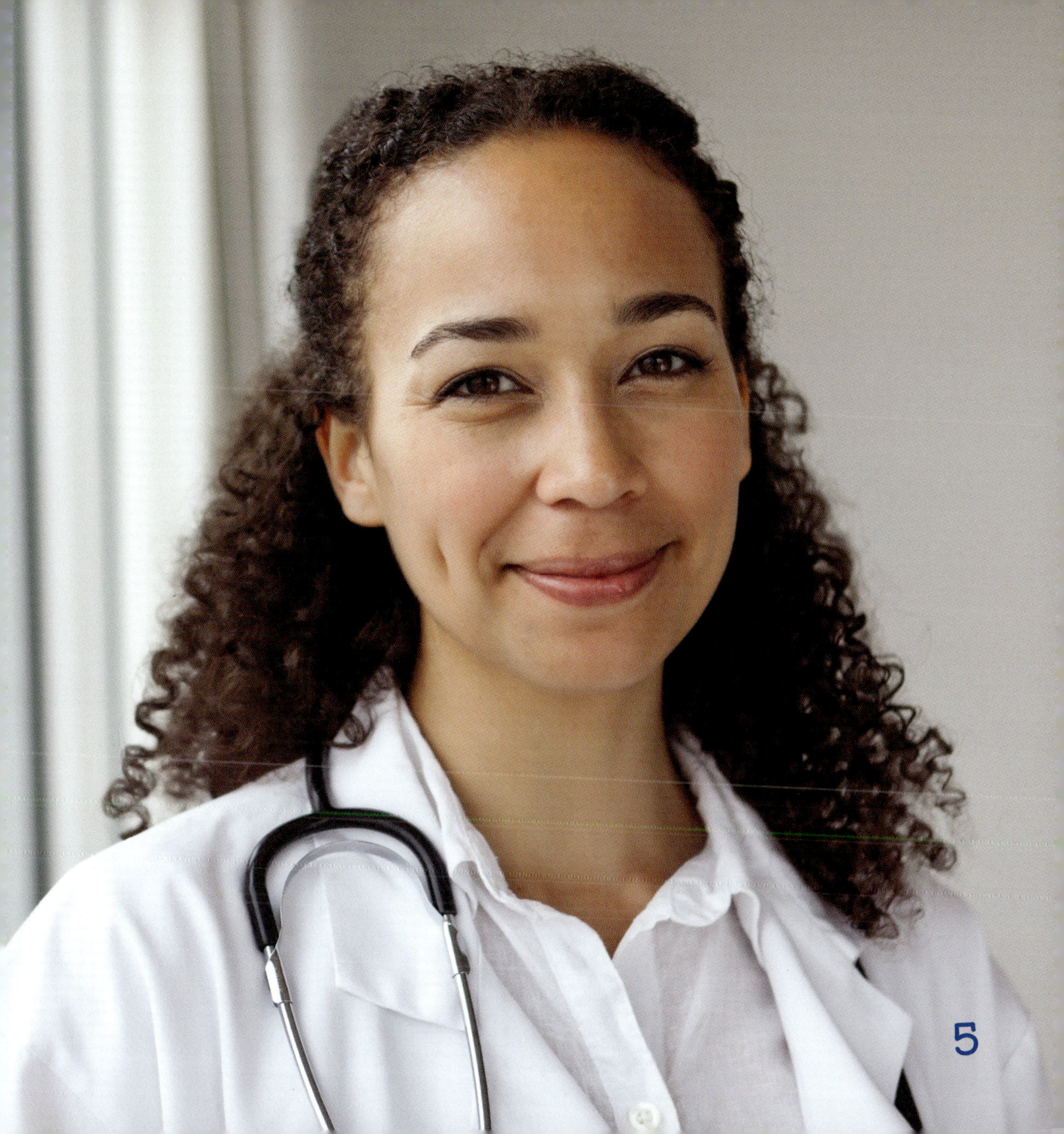

There are many kinds of doctors. Some only see children. Some only see women who are going to have a baby. Many doctors know about **diseases**. Surgeons are doctors who do **operations**. All doctors want to help people stay well.

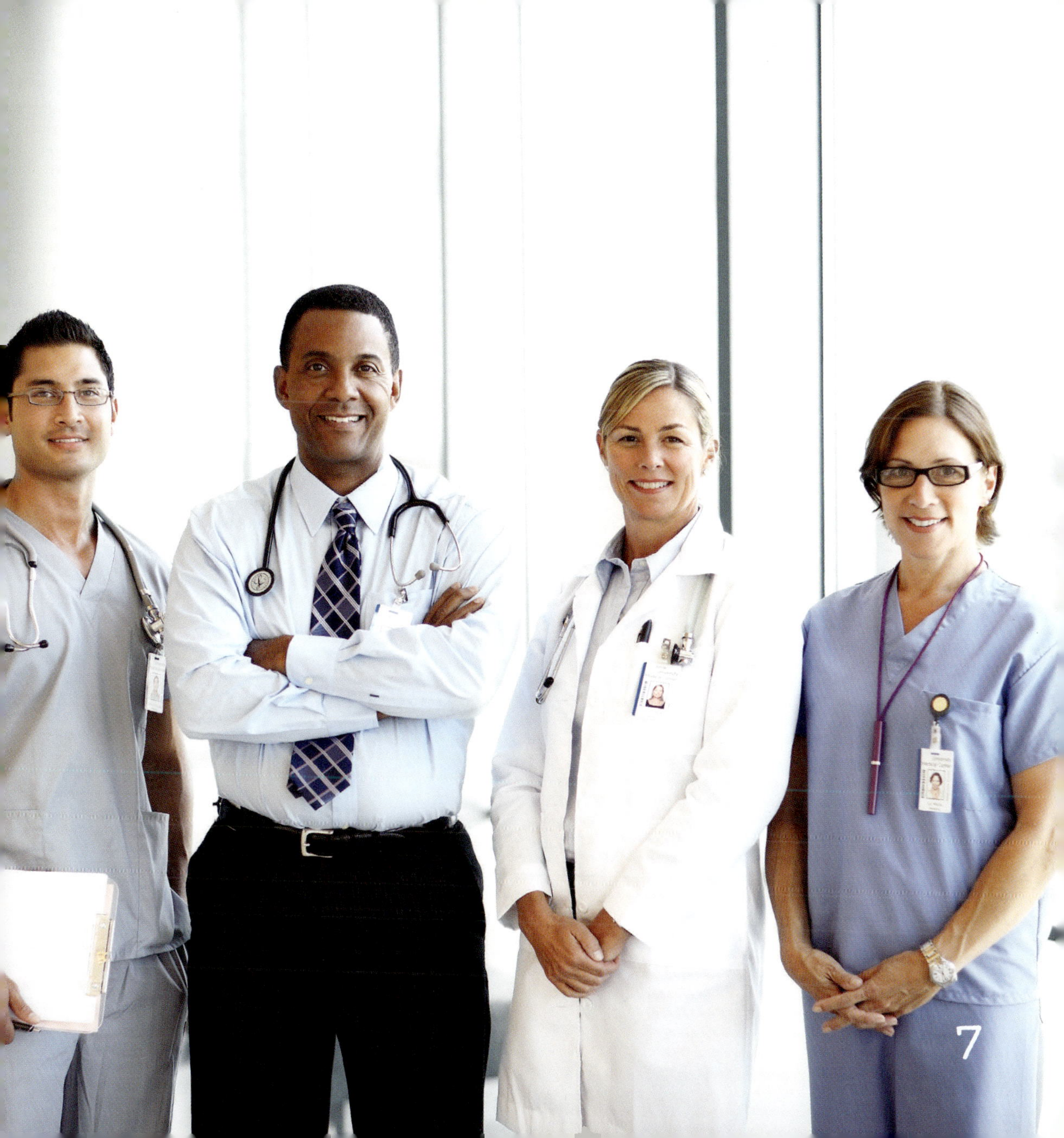

You may go to see your family doctor when you're feeling sick. You may also see this doctor when you're feeling fine. This is called a checkup. Checkups are important. They make sure you're healthy.

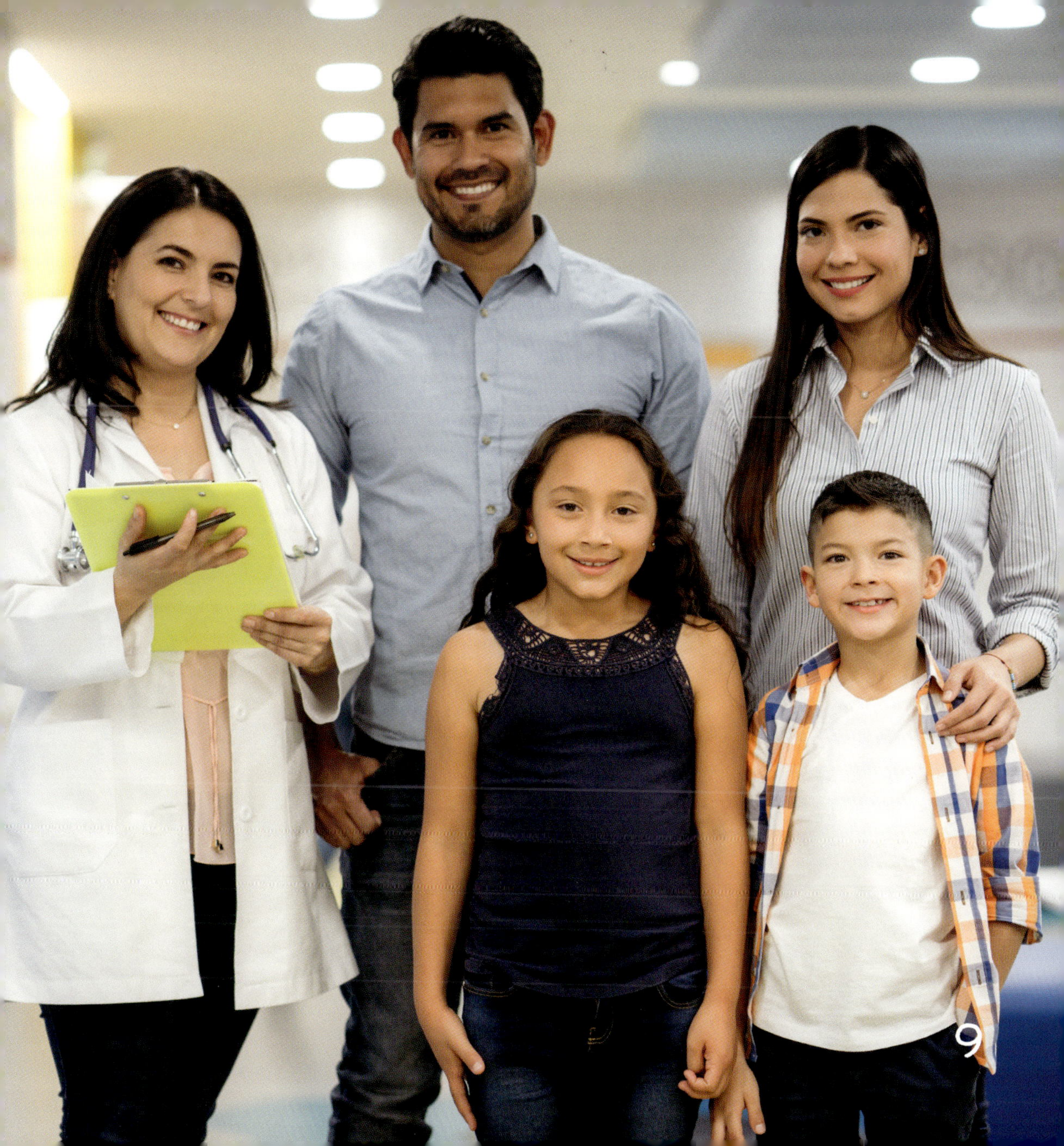

What Do Doctors Do?

When you go for a checkup, you're asked to sit in a room to wait for the doctor. A nurse asks you questions. The nurse sees how tall you are. The nurse also takes your **temperature**.

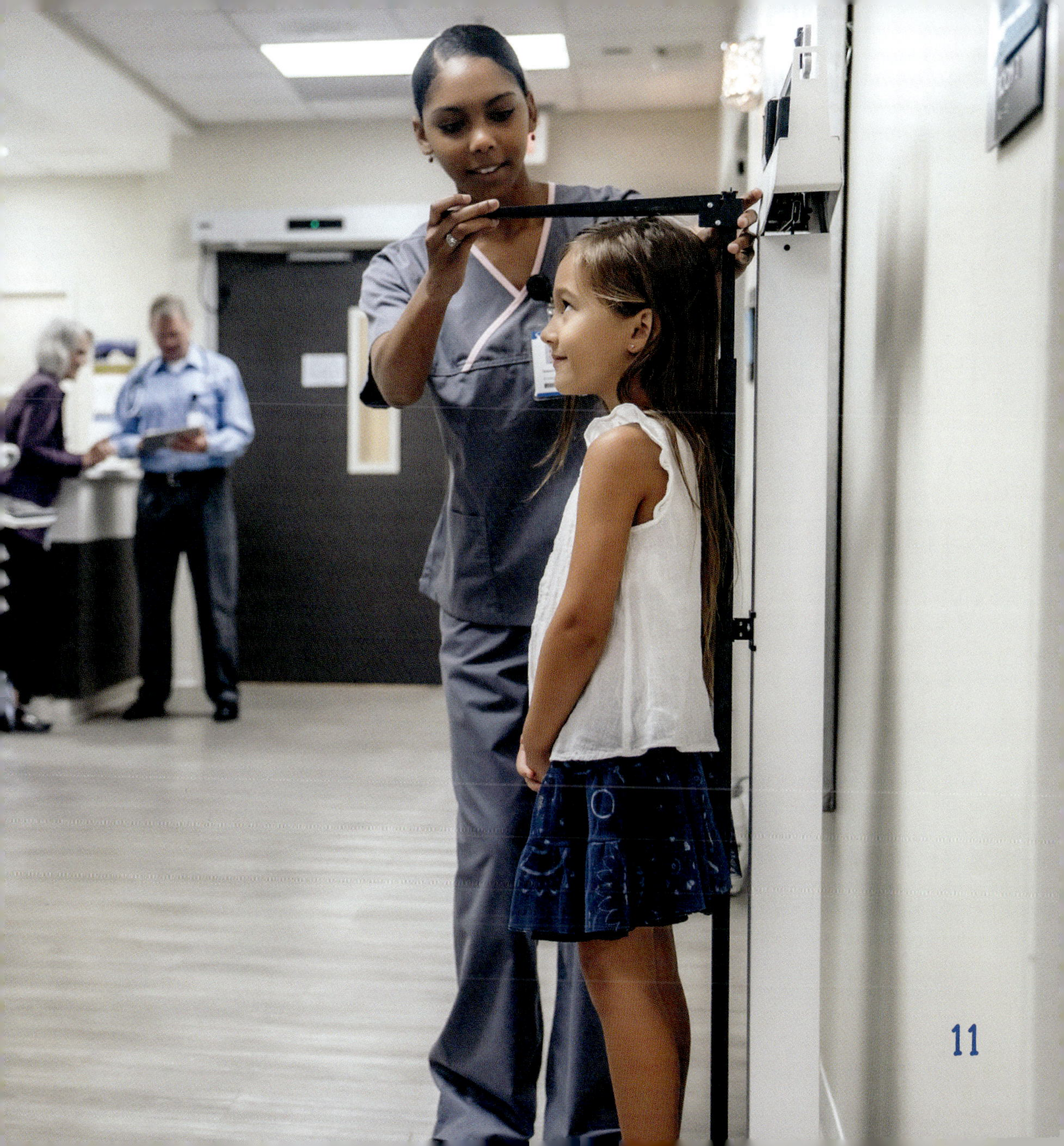

Soon, the doctor comes into the room where you're waiting. The doctor asks you questions too. They also touch your neck, belly, and knees. They do this to make sure you're growing right and nothing hurts.

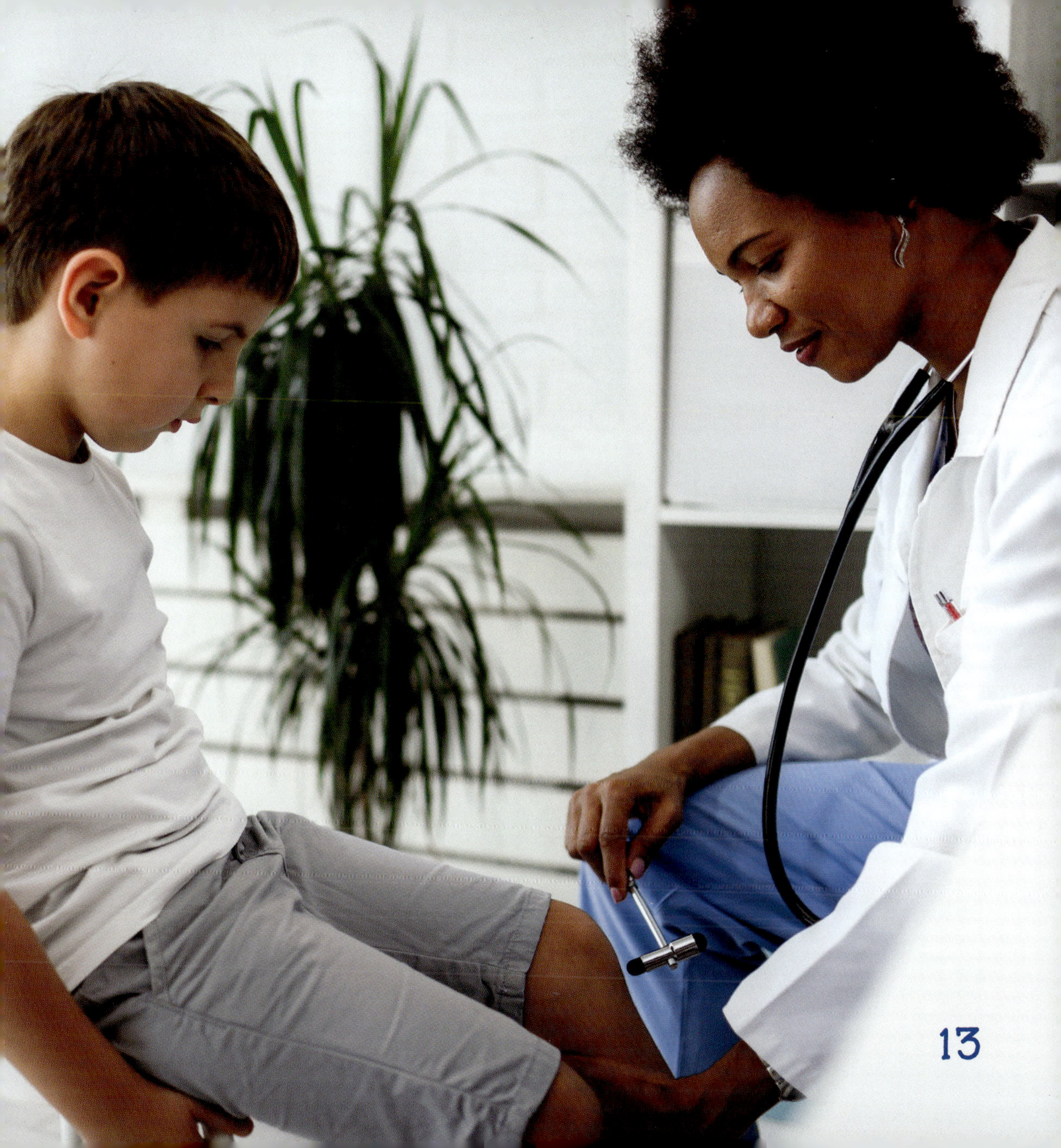

Doctors use special tools to make sure you're healthy. They use a tool to look inside your ears and nose. One tool lets doctors listen to your heart and breathing. Doctors take notes about your health.

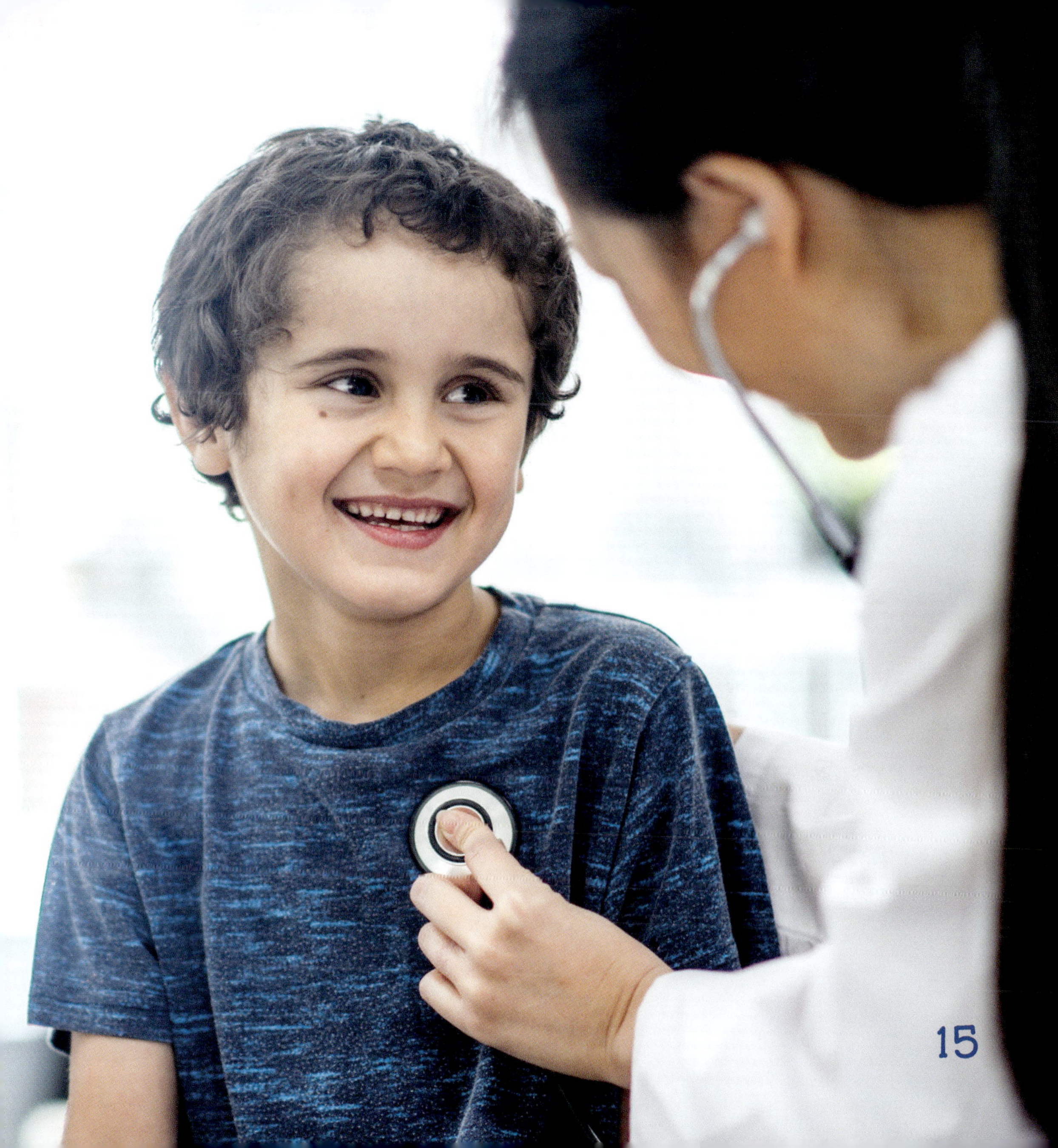

The doctor may give you **medicine**. They may also give you a shot. Shots help keep people from getting sick. Doctors and nurses are very good at giving shots! Some shots hurt a little, but some don't hurt at all.

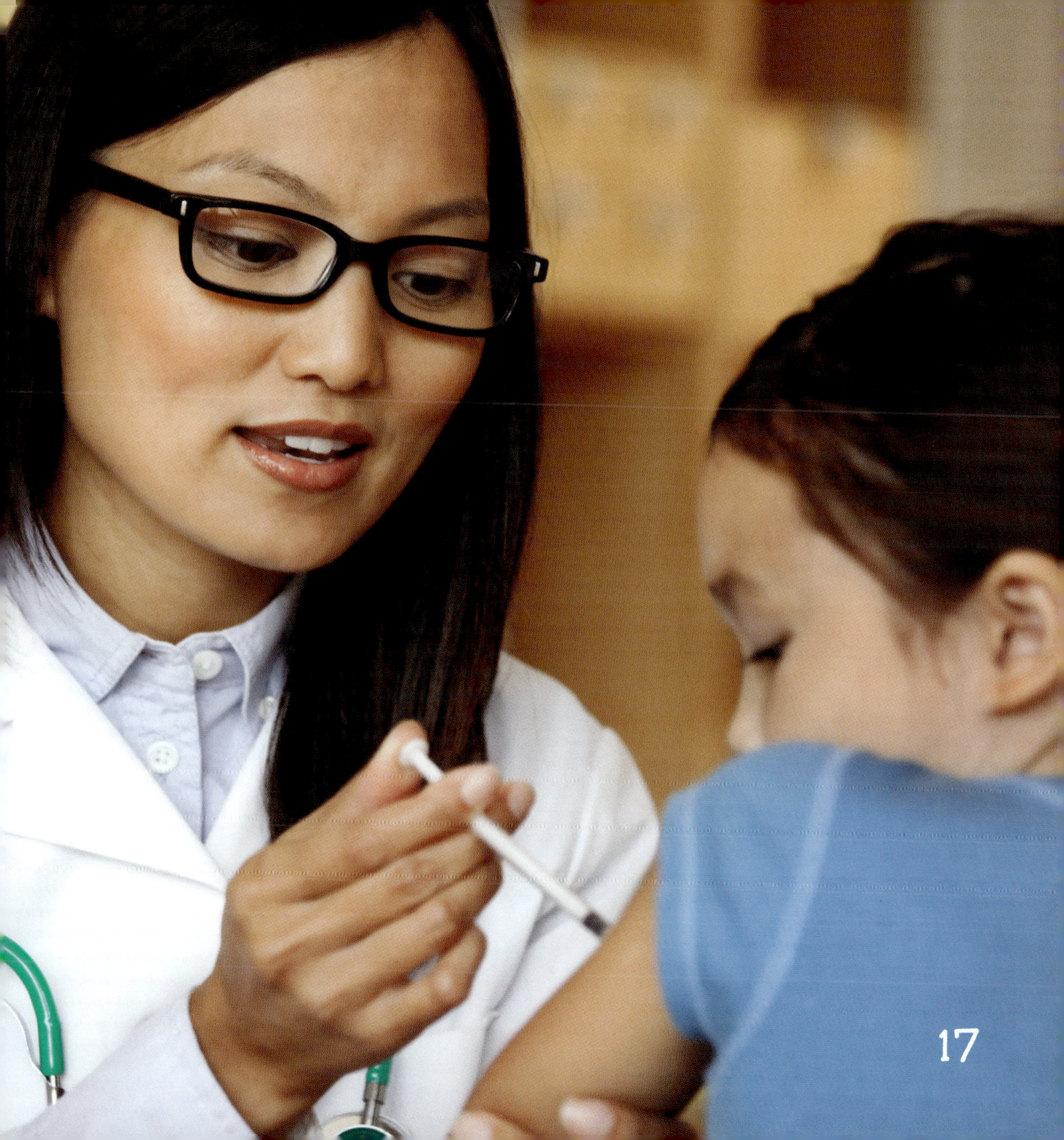

Accidents are things we don't plan on happening. However, they still happen! If you fall off your bike, you may get a bad cut. A doctor can help! Doctors make sure your body heals right after getting hurt.

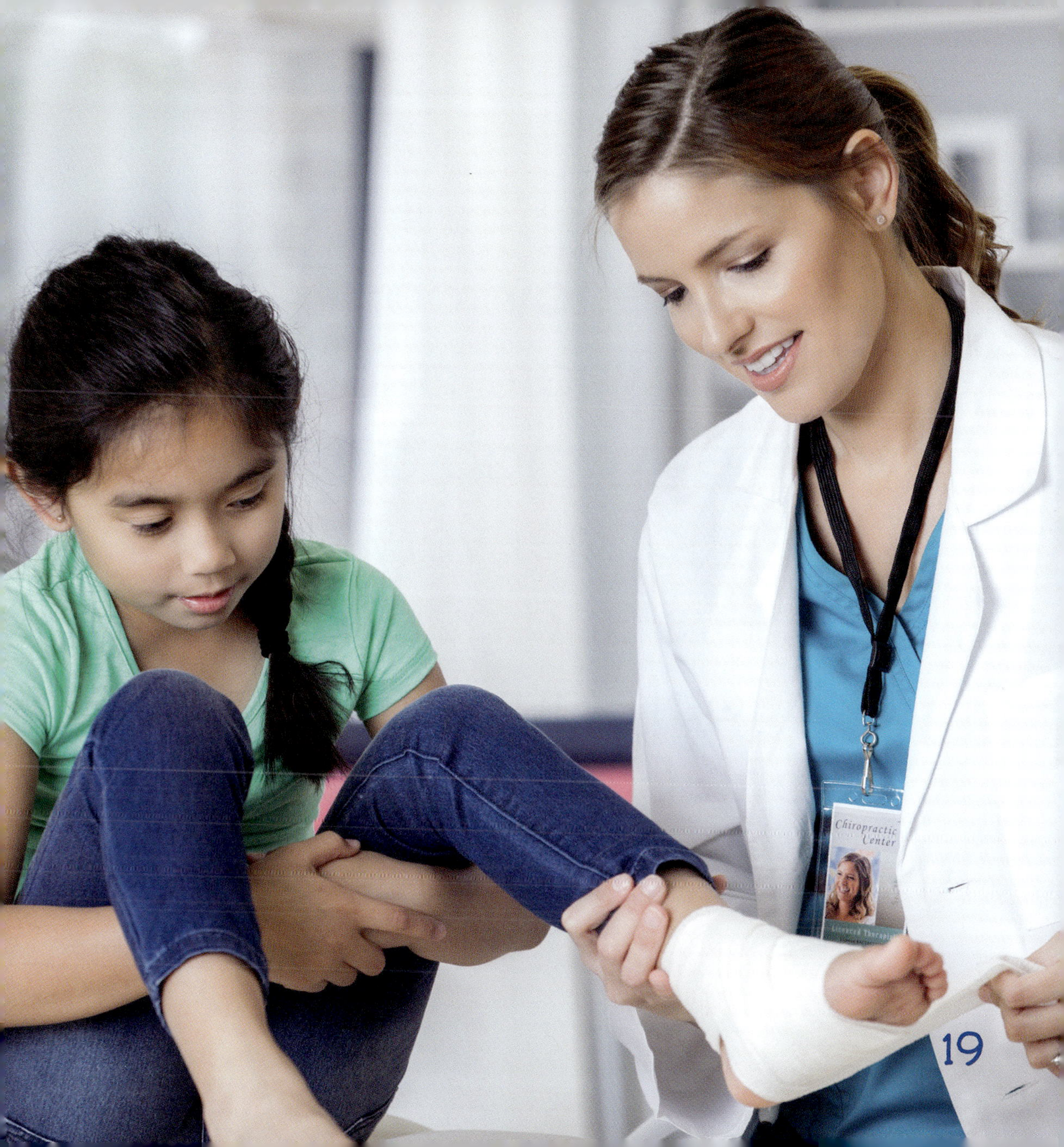
Chiropractic
Center

The **emergency** room (ER) is a place where people go when they've had a bad accident or get very sick. ER doctors and nurses can help people quickly. When someone breaks a bone, they fix it with a cast.

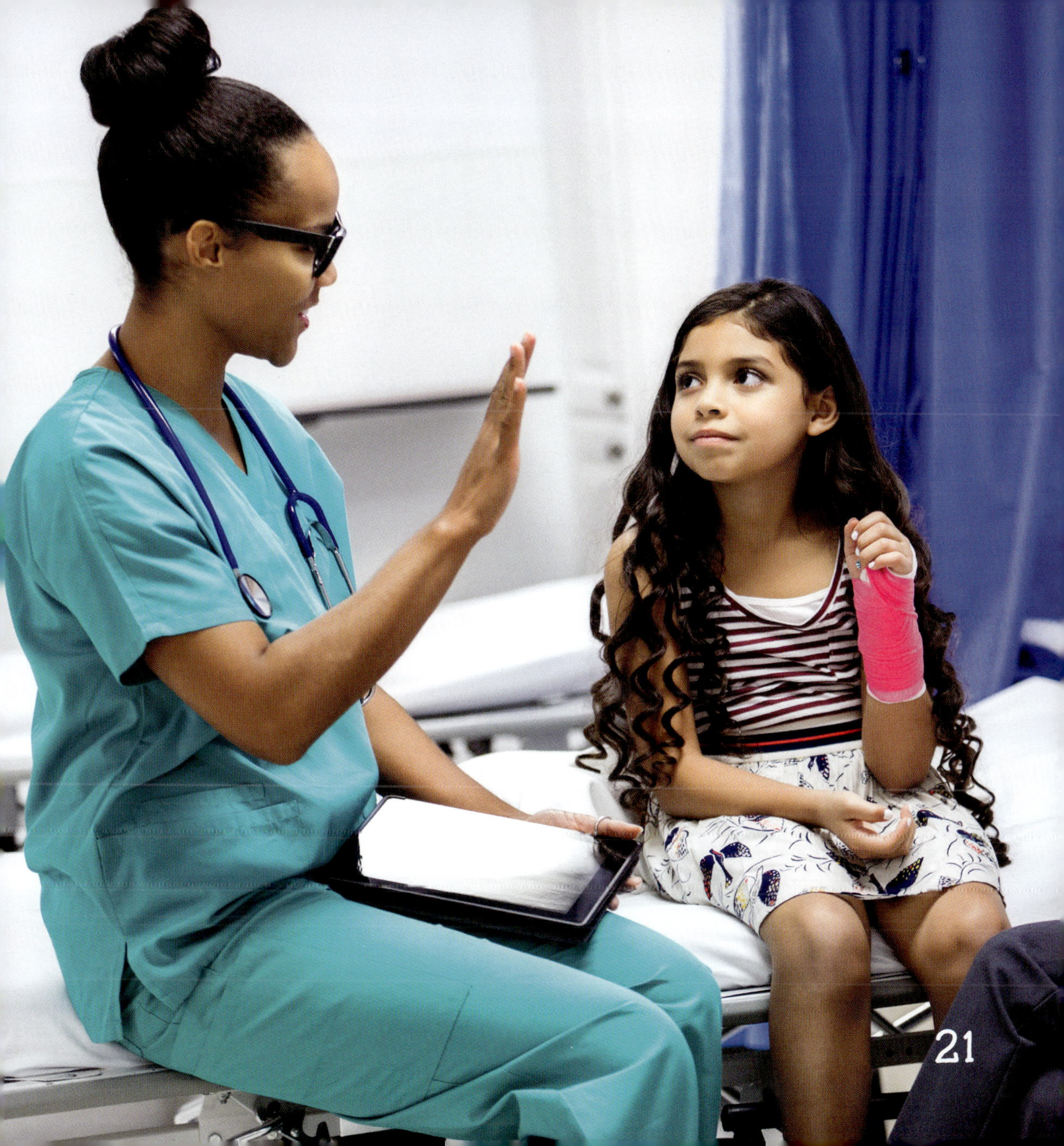

Healthy Bodies

Doctors check our bodies for illnesses and help us when we're hurt. Doctors also help us make healthy choices. They tell us what foods are good for us. They tell us how to stay fit. Doctors want us to be healthy!

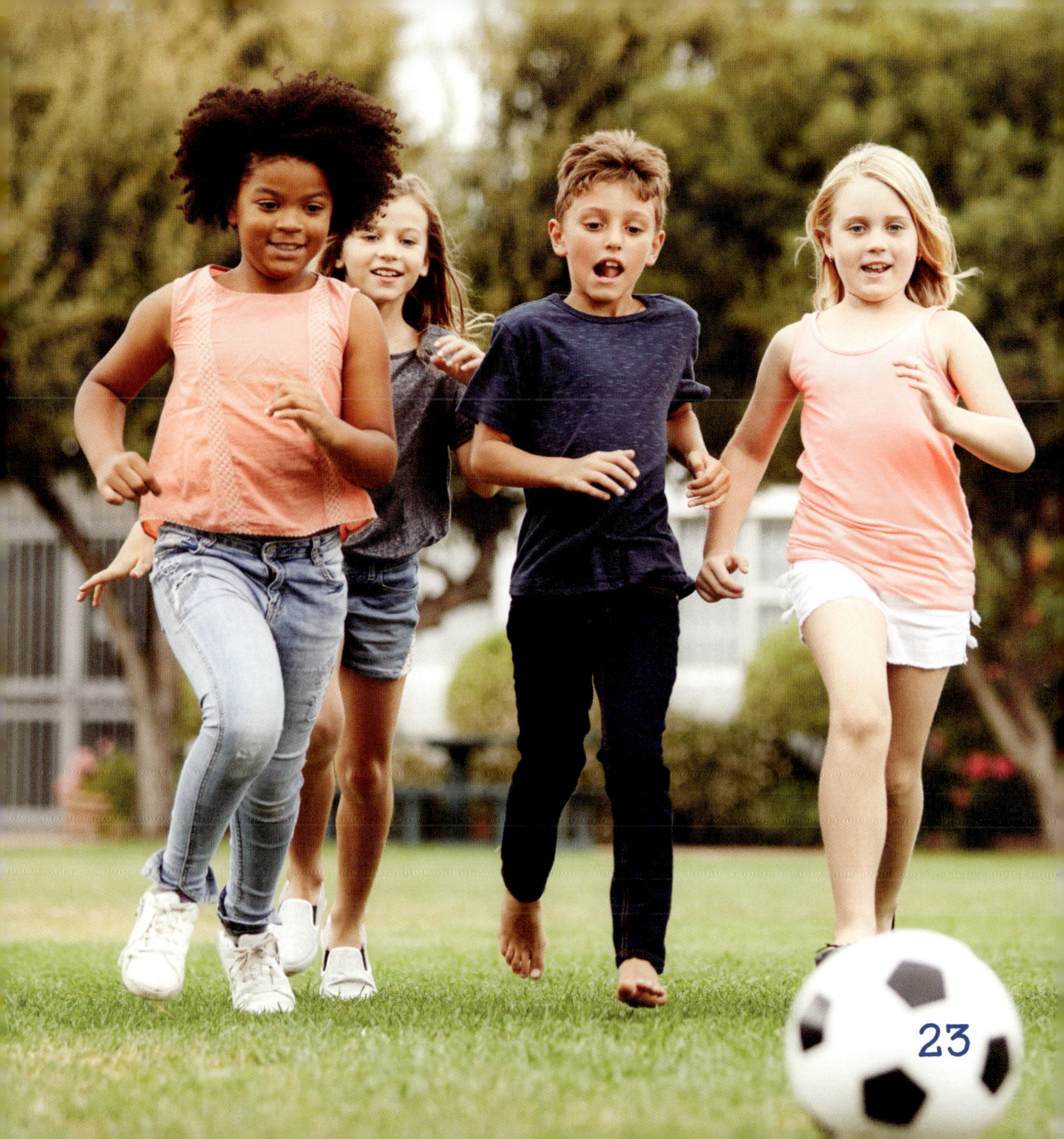

WORDS TO KNOW

diseases: Illnesses of the mind or body.

emergency: A sudden event that requires action right away.

medicine: Something used to stop an illness.

operations: When doctors cut into someone's body in order to fix or take out hurt or sick parts.

temperature: How hot or cold something is.

INDEX